Fabien MEMONG NDENGUE
Dieudonné Davy AMBASSA

Quality of life for Cameroonian prisoners

Fabien MEMONG NDENGUE
Dieudonné Davy AMBASSA

Quality of life for Cameroonian prisoners

An analysis of psychosocial support

ScienciaScripts

Cover image: www.ingimage.com

This book is a translation from the original published under ISBN 978-620-6-72243-4.

Publisher:
Sciencia Scripts
is a trademark of
Dodo Books Indian Ocean Ltd. and OmniScriptum S.R.L publishing group

120 High Road, East Finchley, London, N2 9ED, United Kingdom
Str. Armeneasca 28/1, office 1, Chisinau MD-2012, Republic of Moldova, Europe
Printed at: see last page
ISBN: 978-620-8-09054-8

QUALITY OF LIFE OF CAMEROONIAN PRISONERS: AN ANALYSIS OF PSYCHOSOCIAL SUPPORT

TABLE OF CONTENTS

DEDICATION

A

MARTIAL ZIBI NDENGUE

SUMMARY

Introduction: Our study is entitled: In Cameroon, the prison population is estimated at around 30,000 inmates for a capacity of 9,000, i.e. an occupancy rate of 432% in some prisons such as the Douala Central Prison (OMCT, SOS-torture 2020) [1]. Faced with this overcrowding, prison conditions are becoming inhumane and responsible for the deterioration in the quality of life of prisoners. Prisoners face a brutal break with their support networks. This isolation disrupts family dynamics and generates stress and anxiety. This study raises the problem of the deterioration in the quality of life in an environment that does not allow prisoners to mobilise the resources they need to cope with prison. The adversity of the environment in Cameroon no longer needs to be demonstrated. Inspired by the work of Terra (2003) [2], to reduce suicide, stress and anxiety among prisoners as much as possible, it is necessary to establish a climate of good relations and maintain family ties. Psychosocial support is therefore an essential variable in improving prisoners' quality of life. The aim of this study is therefore to examine the effect of psychosocial support on the quality of life of inmates at Douala Central Prison.

Methodology: A cross-sectional analytical study was carried out in Douala central prison. Data were collected using a questionnaire assessing perceived quality of life and perceived psychosocial support. These tools were chosen on the basis of the literature review we carried out for each of the concepts. The data collected were analysed in two ways: descriptively and differentially. The results of the linear regression analyses reveal that the dimensions of psychosocial support, namely emotional support (**β= .53; p= .001**), esteem support (**β= .44; p= .001**), informational support (**β= .40; p= .001**) and material support (**β= .45; p= .001**) have a statistically significant and positive effect on prisoners' quality of life.

Conclusion: These results clearly indicate that these psychosocial support dimensions could be levers for combating precariousness and improving the quality of life of prisoners in Cameroonian prisons.

Key words: Psychosocial support, Quality of life, Prisoners

INTRODUCTION

Quality of life, which is now the subject of many considerations and growing interest, is a multifactorial and subjective concept. It depends on the conditions in which we live, the personal judgement we make of our own lives and ourselves, and the satisfaction we derive from our own condition. It involves a wide range of physical, psychological and social factors, and extends far beyond the fact of being 'objectively' healthy. Everyone has the right to expect the best possible quality of life, regardless of social, political, geographical or moral difficulties or divisions [3]. The term psychosocial refers to the link between the individual (i.e. his or her reactions, feelings and internal emotional and reasoning processes) and his or her environment, direct surroundings, community and/or culture (i.e. the social context in which he or she lives) [4].

In other words, all people aspire to live in peace and quiet, and this goes beyond the "mere" absence of illness. But then the question is whether prisoners are entitled to enjoy a reasonable quality of life in the same way as other individuals? Is it legitimate to work to improve the condition of prisoners when they have committed criminal and reprehensible acts? ? Is it a priority to alleviate the difficult conditions in prisons and help prisons cope with overcrowding and a lack of resources to fully carry out their custodial and rehabilitation missions?In its 2015 report, Penal Reform International estimated that millions of people around the world are incarcerated and detained in conditions that do not meet international human rights standards. [5]. These prison conditions seriously damage their chances of a productive return to society. For this organisation, the overcrowding of prisons around the world makes it very difficult to apply the minimum standards of detention defined by the United Nations and compromises the health of prisoners. In Cameroon, for example, the prison population is estimated at around 30,000 prisoners for a capacity of of 14,965, with an occupancy rate of 432% in prisons such as Yaoundé Central Prison [1]. The extent to which Cameroon's prisons are prey to worrying overcrowding that does not meet human conditions and international requirements for public detention centres is therefore clear. In this context, the increase in the prison population seems to go hand in hand with a deterioration in prison conditions. It is therefore easy to understand why prisons are regularly criticised for being pathogenic and degrading. The epidemiological data available in the work of Minkoa et al [6] show that 21.3% of inmates at

Yaoundé central prison suffered from suicidal disorders and 33.7% from depressive disorders. Similarly, a study by Eyoum et al [7] found a prevalence of 22.7% of inmates suffering from suicidal disorders in Douala prison. In France, the work of Godin-Blandeau et al [8] shows a very high incidence of numerous pathologies, particularly psychiatric disorders. Nowadays, the purpose of a prison sentence should be to deprive individuals who have broken the law of their freedom, to keep them away from society for the purposes of preserving and protecting citizens, and to prepare, in the long term, for their return to that same society. It is no longer a question of using suffering to atone for one's faults and make amends. In the context of this study, quality of life depends on reception and detention conditions, and proximity to facilitate contact with loved ones. The conditions of detention in our prison system make it impossible to promote factors that protect prisoners' quality of life, because of overcrowding. We believe that the timely and adequate provision of psychosocial support can prevent anxiety and suffering from leading to more serious mental problems, as 33.7% of inmates in Douala central prison suffer from depression, and 22.7% from suicidal ideation, with the associated factors of lack of visits and physical and psychological abuse Eyoum et al [7]. We therefore thought it appropriate to conduct a study on the impact of of psychosocial support on the quality of life of inmates at Douala Central Prison.

1. STUDY QUESTIONS

1.1 General question

Does psychosocial support improve the quality of life of inmates at Douala Central Prison?

1.2 Specific questions

❖ What is the quality of life like for inmates at Douala Central Prison?

❖ What is the perceived psychosocial support for the quality of life of inmates at Douala Central Prison?

❖ What is the link between psychosocial support and the quality of life of inmates at Douala Central Prison?

2. RESEARCH HYPOTHESES

2.1. General research hypotheses

Psychosocial support would improve the quality of life of inmates at Douala Central Prison.

2.2. Operational research hypotheses

These hypotheses were formulated on the basis of the operationalisation of the independent variable (psychosocial support) into four dimensions following House's model (1981) [9]. Following this operationalisation, four hypotheses were formulated:

❖ HO1: Psychosocial support focusing on emotional support would increase the quality of life of inmates at Douala Central Prison

❖ HO2: psychosocial support focusing on esteem support would increase the quality of life of prisoners in Douala central prison.

❖ HO3: Psychosocial support focusing on informative support would increase the quality of life of inmates at Douala Central Prison.

❖HO4 : Psychosocial support focused on material support would increase the quality of life of inmates at Douala Central Prison.

3. AIMS OF THE STUDY

3.1. General objective

Studying the effect of psychosocial support on the quality of life of inmates at Douala Central Prison

1.2 Specific objectives

❖ Measuring the quality of life of inmates at Douala Central Prison.

❖ Determining the quality of psychosocial support for prisoners in Douala Central Prison

❖ Researching an association between perceived psychosocial support and quality of life among inmates of Douala Central Prison

CHAPTER I
LITERATURE REVIEW

To gain a better understanding of this theme, the key concepts of psychosocial support, quality of life and prison will be analysed.

Generally speaking, individuals show a number of normal reactions to unusual events, including the following aspects and their manifestations:

- Emotional: Anxiety, grief, guilt, anger, irritability, frustration, sadness, shame, indifference, loss of hope, loss of meaning, feelings of emptiness;
- Mental: Lack of concentration, memory loss, confusion, intrusive thoughts, difficulty making decisions, disorganised thoughts;
- Physical symptoms. Increased heart rate, trouble sleeping, aches and pains (stomach, head), back and neck pain, muscle tremors and tension, loss of energy, inability to rest and relax;
- Social. Risk-taking, over- or under-eating, increased alcohol or cigarette consumption, aggression, withdrawal, isolation.

In fact, the reactions described may be the result of somatisation following a traumatic event that caused a break with the mainstream of life. This study focuses on people who have experienced a break with their home environment, imprisonment, loss of freedom and the shock of a trial. In fact, the work of Memong Ndengue (2022) [10] has shown that the shock of imprisonment, the shock of the trial, added to the conditions of detention, which are not the best in Cameroon, contribute to increasing the suffering of detainees. In fact, as many epidemiological studies have shown, the suffering of prisoners leads to mental problems such as depression, affective and mood disorders and suicidal disorders. Eyoum et al [7] The conditions of detention in the Cameroonian penitentiary system do not make it possible to promote factors that protect the quality of life of prisoners, due to prison overcrowding, the deterioration of premises and the long wait for the outcome of trials. The aim of this chapter is to summarise the literature on quality of life in prisons in Cameroon. in general and on the quality of prisoners in particular. We will also present the notion of psychosocial support.

I - 1 Psychosocial support

The term "psychosocial" refers to the dynamic relationship between the psychological and social facets of a person, which influence each other. The psychological facet includes emotional and rational processes, feelings and reactions. The social facet includes relationships, family and community networks, social values and cultural practices. Psychosocial support" refers to actions that respond to the psychological and social needs of individuals, families and communities. It is widely accepted that we provide psychosocial support to help people who have suffered a crisis to recover. Provided in a timely and appropriate manner, this support to the prisoners in this study can prevent anxiety and suffering from leading to more serious mental problems in the prisoners.

I - 1.1 History, Concept and Measures

The role of social relationships and their contribution to well-being and health has been the subject of reflection and study for over a century. In 1897, Durkheim postulated that breakdowns in social ties led to a loss of social resources and a weakening of social roles and norms. His study of suicide showed that it was more prevalent among individuals with fewer social ties, particularly prisoners. [11] The first social ecologists (Park & Burgess, 1926) [12] also noted an increase in behavioural problems in uprooted populations.

I - 1.2 Support functions

For Orford (1992) [13] support functions are defined as various aspects related to the quality of relationships or the capacity of relationships to fulfil different support functions. It refers to the concrete help that the entourage provides to an individual or group of individuals going through a difficult situation. This dimension of support refers to the actual use of social support resources (Tardy, 1985) [14] This active support can take the form of listening, expressing concerns, lending money, helping with a task, hearing the opinion of others, or showing affection. For Barrera (1981) [15], this type of support is the set of actions that provide concrete help to the person. The literature identifies the main functions of social support (Cohen and Wills, 1985; Jacobson, 1986; Leavy, 1983; Orford, 1992; Wills, 1985): affective, material, cognitive, normative and socialisation support. [16] In the context of this study, quality of life depends on reception and detention conditions: limited-capacity facilities, close proximity to facilitate contact with relatives. The conditions of detention in the Cameroonian penitentiary system do not allow for the promotion of protective factors, nor of health, let alone quality of life, due to overcrowding. The idea of strengthening a social support network for prisoners is vital because its role here is to help people who have suffered a crisis to recover. Provided at the right time and in the right way, this support can prevent anxiety and suffering giving rise to more serious mental problems in Cameroonian prisoners, as described by eyoum et al (2023). [7] This type of support is the set of actions that provide concrete help to the person in prison and help them to cope with the shock of confinement, the shock of the prison environment, the break with their home environment,the shock of the trial and the shock of the act that landed him in prison. [17]. The health of prisoners, whether mental or physical, is central to their quality of life, and its protection depends on the living environment. According to the World Health Organisation, an inclusive community is a key determinant of mental health through its protective role and social support, i.e. knowing that you are loved, valued and part of a social network has a very positive influence on physical and mental health (WHO, 2014). [18] According to the work of Bruchon-Schweitser (2002), [19] these various types of support must be considered not only according to their function, but also according to how well they match the stressful situation and the individual's expectations and needs. Moreover, this author stresses that receiver satisfaction depends on consistency between the type of support and the source of support (family, friends, colleague, etc.). Psychosocial support is recognised as having an impact on prisoners' lives, particularly their mental health. In order to reduce suicide, stress and anxiety among prisoners as much as possible, it is necessary to establish a climate of good relations and maintain family ties. Terra (2003) [2] Psychosocial support is therefore an essential variable in improving prisoners' mental health.

This support is a powerful stress moderator, and plays a protective role, especially in a context of social isolation such as prison. The person is facing a break with their home environment. They need a professional who will listen and communicate constructively. But unfortunately this is not the case in our prisons. Although humanisation involves listening, speaking, touching and looking, these four concepts are not given much consideration in the treatment of prisoners. The look remains that of surveillance, the touch which is the common denominator is the search, the tone is always threatening and intimidating, (ex inmates of Kondengui 2017). The results of the correlation analysis of the study on psychosocial support and the mental health of inmates in Bafia main prison in Cameroon showed that the dimensions of perceived psychosocial support have a significant and positive relationship with perceived mental health. Memong (2022) [10]

I - 1.3 Research establishing links between social support and health

This section presents research linking social support and health, which is an important facet of quality of life. Health is a state of complete physical, mental and social well-being and not merely the absence of disease or infirmity (WHO 1946). [20] This definition gives an overview of the concept of health, suggesting that talking about good health among prisoners is an approach that integrates biological, psychological and social aspects.

I - 1.3.1 Poor people

All epidemiological studies agree that low-income populations are the most vulnerable when it comes to mental health. Socio-economic status is considered to be the best predictor of mental health. In fact, around 30% of these populations experience psychological distress at any given time, and they make up the majority of people receiving mental health services. However, numerous studies, such as those by Tousignant and Caron (2005) [21], point to a lack of available social support in low-income populations, as in the case of prisoners.

I - 1.3.2 Depressive populations

Perceived and received support has been studied in relation to depression. A low level of social support is associated with the development of a major depressive episode (Wade & Kendler, 2000) [22]. According to the study by MINKOA et al (2020) [7], the Cameroonian prison population faces enormous stress.

I - 1.3.3 Negative social interactions

Positive social support can help reduce the negative impact of various stressors on mental health. Conversely, negative social interactions with peers can exacerbate mental health problems, as is the case in prisons. The theoretical stress buffering model is the most comprehensive and widely studied model of social support in relation to health (Lakey & Cohen, 2000) [23].

In short, social support is an excellent tool for intervention and community action. It makes it possible to take account of the link between the individual and the collective because it is at the crossroads of a traditional approach marked by concern for personal factors and a community approach based on the social environment. According to Boucher and Laprise (2004, p. 118) [24], social support is "a complex phenomenon that enables individuals, groups and communities to give and receive, to feel the benefits of a range of gestures and assistance from close and wider circles". In other words, it is a social resource that can be mobilised by a group of people in the same situation to cope with life's difficulties. Studies in Cameroonian prisons do not abound in the literature, which allows us to highlight a specific context for the benefits of this support among prisoners in the Douala Central Prison.

I - 2. Quality of life

I - 2.1 History and definition

The term "quality of life" is relatively new to our vocabulary. It made its first official appearance in 1964, in a presidential speech by London B. Johnson (Shea and King-Farlow, 1976) [25]. Subsequently, this new concern for the quality of life of Americans was taken up in scientific circles. Initially, quality of life was closely associated with the evaluation of the quality of the physical environment, the neighbourhood and the community on the basis of statistical data, considered to be "social indicators" [26] (Carlisle, 1972; Duncan, 1969; Hoffenberg, 1970; Sawhill, 1969; USDHEW; 1969). Quality of life is assessed on the basis of a It is based on a number of objective indicators, usually statistical, and relates to groups of people or environments. Today, empirical research and theoretical reflection are attempting to identify the factors responsible for quality of life. On the one hand, authors are proposing frameworks for analysing what constitutes quality of life. Bubolz (1980) [27] proposes an ecological model. For Reich and Zautra (1984) [28] quality of life is about the control one has over one's life. Bigelow et al (1982) [29] suggest instead that quality of life is about striking the right balance between needs and resources (personal and social), role performance and environmental expectations. In parallel with this theoretical approach, empirical research is examining the role of psychological variables (Abbey & Andrews, 1985) [30] in people's perception of their quality of life. In short, quality of life has been a fashionable concept for the last fifteen years or so, and it has succeeded in supplanting and integrating competing notions (well-being, health, life satisfaction, happiness, etc.). And yet, even if it seems banal and obvious, it is a protean and even polysemous concept that is difficult to define and delimit. Indeed, there can be very different conceptions of quality of life, depending on whether we focus on objective aspects such as living conditions, or subjective aspects such as happiness or satisfaction, or on physical components (organic health) and mental components (psychological health).

I - 2.2 Quality of life indicators for prisoners

This notion has been under-explored in scientific studies carried out in Cameroonian prisons, but is well protected by the laws governing judicial detention.

I - 2.2.1 Prisoners' health

The right to health is fundamental and indispensable to the exercise of many other rights. It concerns not only the right to benefit from appropriate and timely medical care, but also the management of the factors that affect health. These include the right to food and nutrition, access to safe drinking water and adequate sanitation, the right to clothing and housing, and the right to breathe fresh air and engage in physical and mental exercise. While people all over the world are confronted with inequality of treatment when it comes to health (BOUOPDA 2021), [31] the effects of poverty and deprivation of liberty combine to deny prisoners' right to health. There is no other place where access to medicine and the means to lead a healthy life are more neglected than behind prison walls, where disease is the most common cause of death.

I - 2.2.2 Physical and personal safety of prisoners

In principle, when an individual's actions transgress the laws of society, the application of a custodial sentence is the responsibility of the judiciary in order to bring the person back into line. However, if a person is deprived of their liberty, it is the responsibility of the State to ensure that their fundamental rights are respected. The United Nations Human Rights Committee considers this responsibility to be an obligation on States to protect the rights of people made vulnerable by their status as persons deprived of their liberty. Prisoners must benefit from the right to protection, which is fundamental for them in relation to state institutions. Indeed, article 10 of the United Nations International Covenant on Civil and Political Rights requires that prisoners be treated "with humanity and respect for the inherent dignity of the human person". However, if we look at society as a whole, we see that it is increasingly driven by a single imperative, which some see as being implemented through fear: "to increase the severity of punishment for offenders and deviants, to increase sentences, to lengthen them, to make them ever harsher and more humiliating in the hope that they will act as a deterrent".

I - 2.2.3 Prison environment

These are the geographical living conditions, the immediate environment in which prisoners develop their vitality. Studies have shown that, as a result of their living environment, detainees lose a certain number of skills (language, behaviour, intellectual activities, protection and resistance-related disabilities) and social abilities, as well as their ability to look after and care for themselves, which is evidence of the deterioration in their quality of life. (Handicap International, 2012) [32]. In principle, detention should not aggravate the suffering caused by deprivation of liberty, as prison and detention conditions have a considerable impact on the health, well-being and quality of life of detainees (Nelson Minimum Rules 2015) [33].

I - 3 Prison

According to the Office of the United Nations High Commissioner for Human Rights (2004), [22] [34] Prisons have existed in most societies for centuries. They are usually used to incarcerate individuals until they are brought before a judicial body. They may be awaiting trial, the execution of a judgement, a sentence of exile or the payment of bail, a fine or a debt. Prison can also be used to deprive people of their freedom for a long time if they have posed a particular threat to a particular regime or leader. The use of imprisonment as an immediate court-ordered punishment was adopted in Western Europe and North America in the 18th century. It gradually spread to most countries, often as a manifestation of colonial oppression. Over the years, the purpose of imprisonment has given rise to considerable controversy, which continues today. For some, it should be used exclusively to punish wrongdoers; others argue that its main purpose is to deter both those in prison from committing further offences and those who do. on release, than those who might have a propensity to commit a crime. Another view is that the purpose of incarcerating individuals is to reform or rehabilitate them. In other words, once they are in prison, they will come to recognise the error of their criminal behaviour and acquire the skills that will enable them to lead a law-abiding life once they are released. Sometimes people are rehabilitated through work. In some cases, people may be imprisoned because the offence they have committed proves that they are a serious danger to public safety. In practice, the objectives of imprisonment will be interpreted as a combination of all or some of these justifications, the particular mix of which will depend on the circumstances of each individual prisoner. There is a growing view that imprisonment is an expensive last resort that should only be used when the inadequacy of a non-custodial sentence is clear to the court.

I - 3.1 Organisation and operation of prisons in Cameroon

I - 3.1.1 Situation of prisons in Cameroon

Prison life is governed by a number of international, regional and national legislative texts. Some of these instruments are of a general nature and derive mainly from treaties that apply to prisons by inference, while others are more specific and serve as tools for the direct, day-to-day management of the environment in which prisoners live. To get an idea of the prison environment, a detailed look at the buildings and infrastructure as well as at all the inmates provides clear indications for any uncompromising analysis. Buildings and infrastructure The state of affairs in Cameroon's prisons shows that the infrastructure has deteriorated badly, and that the capacity of the prisons has been greatly exceeded.

I - 3.1.2. State of prison structures

Buildings intended to house prisoners must have the characteristics set out in No. 9 of the set of minimum rules. These include cells, dormitories, sanitary and electrical installations, ventilation and hygiene (minimum rules for detention). However, according to a report by (ACAT, December 2014 ACAT (Action by Christians for the Abolition of Torture). [34] the prison system in Cameroon has many shortcomings and there is reason to believe that none of the above provisions are fully respected. Indeed, the ageing infrastructure means that prisons today are a world apart, where minimum living conditions are hard to find. From this point of view, it is well known that most of Cameroon's prison infrastructure is in a state of serious disrepair, as it is made up of old buildings, some of which date back to the colonial period and have not been visibly maintained, let alone renovated, for ages, following the example of the Bafoussam and Yoko prisons, built in 1952, and the Douala prison in 1930. Such a situation is at odds with the terms of the minimum rules, particularly with regard to point 10, which states: "Detention premises and, in particular, those intended for the accommodation of prisoners during the night, shall meet the requirements of hygiene, having regard to the climate, particularly as regards air cubic capacity, minimum surface area, lighting, heating and ventilation" [33]. Point 11 states that "in any premises where prisoners are required to live or work:Windows must be large enough to allow prisoners to read and work in natural light; the layout of these windows must allow fresh air to enter, whether or not there is artificial ventilation. Artificial light shall be sufficient to enable the prisoner t o read or work without impairing his sight". Point 12 also states that "sanitary facilities shall be such as to enable the prisoner to satisfy his natural needs at the proper time, in a clean and decent manner". Also for the comfort of the Point 13 states that "Bathing and showering facilities shall be sufficient to enable and require every prisoner to use them, at a temperature appropriate to the climate and as frequently as is necessary for general hygiene according to the season and geographical area, but at least once a week in a temperate climate", while point 14 stresses that "All premises regularly used by prisoners shall be kept in a perfect state of maintenance and cleanliness". From the above, if we look at the prison environment in Cameroon, we see a huge gap between standards and reality. Criticism is constantly levelled at the precarious state of the infrastructure and inadequate architecture. In many cases, for example, the electricity network is inadequate, in addition to the distribution of drinking water and the communications system, which date from a distant era. [33]

I - 3.1.3. Prison population

On 31 August 2000, 19,691 people were incarcerated in Cameroon's prisons. In April 2003, the prison population stood at 20,273, while in March 2005 it was 22,098. In July 2010, the prison population stood at 24,238 inmates for a capacity of 17,000 spread across 74 operational prisons, including 10 central, 48 main, and 16 secondary. ACAT (December 2014). [34] This figure is set to rise, as in 2020 the prison population is estimated to be around 30,000 inmates for a capacity of 14,965, i.e. an occupancy rate of around 432% in the central prisons of Yaoundé and Douala (OMCT, SOS-torture 2020). [1] Prisons hold three categories of people: those on remand, those who have been convicted and those held in police custody.At the national level, article 20 of Decree no. 92/052 of 27 March 1992 on the organisation of the penitentiary system in Cameroon, and article 553 of the Code of Criminal Procedure, require a strict separation between remand prisoners, convicted prisoners, women and minors. In the case of minors, the Article 706 paragraph 1 of the Code of Criminal Procedure states that "a minor may only be detained in a re-education establishment or in a special section of a prison authorised to hold minors". Paragraph 2 goes on to state that: "in the absence of a re-education establishment or special section, a minor may be detained in a prison for adults, but must be separated from them", Article 706(2). [35] The situations prevailing in Cameroon are therefore in violation of established international standards and have a significant impact on human rights protection policies. This is illustrated in almost all of Cameroon's main prisons. In this respect, the cohabitation of minors with other categories of detainees, for example, is not conducive to their re-education as provided for in the United Nations Rules for the Protection of Juveniles Deprived of their Liberty or the Code of Criminal Procedure, which prioritises the social reintegration of minors; this reintegration stems from the education they receive in a prison designed to re-socialise them rather than condemn them. On a day-to-day basis, this cohabitation is likely to accentuate their delinquency insofar as they are subject to all kinds of violations by adults.

Pre-trial detention is the temporary deprivation of liberty of a person prosecuted for an offence that he or she is alleged to have committed. It is limited in time, according to article 218 of the Code of Criminal Procedure. It is an exceptional measure that can only be ordered in the event of a crime, and article 221 states that "the duration of pre-trial detention is set by the investigating judge in the warrant. It may not exceed 6 months [36]. However, it may be extended by reasoned order for a maximum of 12 months in the case of a felony and 6 months in the case of a misdemeanour". Unfortunately, there are prisoners whose stay in prison has far exceeded the limits provided for by this legal framework, and analyses link this violation to an infringement of the presumption of innocence. Observation shows that abusive pre-trial detention is one of the main causes of overcrowding in Cameroon's prisons.

Table 1: Some studies in prisons in Cameroon

Authors	Country	Website study	Results
Minkoa Ngah et al (2020)	Cameroon	Central Prison Yaoundé	21.3% of inmates at Yaoundé Central Prison suffered from suicidal and depressive disorders(33,7%).
Memong Ndengue, F. et al (2024).	Cameroon	Bafia main prison	Show that perceived mental health has a significant and positive relationship with each of the dimensions of psychosocial support among inmates of the main prison in Bafia. Perceived emotional support (r= 0, 30; p<.01) ; Esteem support (r= 0.31; p<.01),Perceived informational support(r= 0.33; p<.01), Perceived material support (r= 0.18; p<.05).
Christian EYOUM et al (2023)	Cameroon	Prison Douala power station	A prevalence of 22,7% of prisoners suffering from suicidal disorders in Douala prison.

CHAPTER II
MATERIALS AND METHODS

II - 1 Type of study

This study was cross-sectional and analytical

II - 2 Study site

The study will take place at the Douala Central Prison in Cameroon, which is one of the most overcrowded prisons in the country. The prison was established in 1911 and has a capacity of around 800 places, with over 4,000 inmates to date. In addition to the observations made at the site, it was also chosen because of its proximity to the study. In fact, given that this research is being carried out as part of a Master's degree at the University of Douala, the Douala site was also chosen because it would limit travel and the expenses associated with deployment in the field.

II - 3. period and duration of the study

This study took place from June 2023 to April 2024, i.e. 10 months. Data collection took place in December 2023.

II - 4 Study population

It comprised all inmates of Douala Central Prison Inclusion criteria

➢ be detained in Douala Central Prison and present during the investigation period

➢ Be able to communicate and respond to interviews. This selection will be based on the level of study of the inmates, their consent to take part in the research, etc.

Non-inclusion criteria

➢ Be detained in Douala Central Prison and be a minor

➢ Being on free duty or secondment

➢ Be unable to communicate and answer our questionnaire Exclusion criteria

➢ Any questionnaire not completed

➢ Any questionnaire bearing an identity (name, telephone number)

II - 5 Sampling

We used non-probability convenience sampling.

II - 6 Sample size

This study covered a **total of 700 prisoners** who received the questionnaire. After counting the responses, **421 prisoners were** selected according to the selection criteria.

II - 7 Materials and methods II - 7.1. Methods

The analysis methods used were as follows:

- Administrative procedures

- Technical procedures

II - 7.1.1 Administrative procedures

This study began with the drafting of the protocol, which was validated by the dissertation director and then by the faculty. Next, an ethical clearance was obtained from the Institutional Ethics Committee of the University of Douala, and an authorisation to collect data was obtained from the regional delegate of the penitentiary administration of the littoral.

II. 7.1.2 The independent variable

According to Myers & Hansen (2007), [37] the independent variable is a variable that the researcher manipulates voluntarily. It is also the causal variable. It is independent because it does not depend on another variable.
The independent variable in our study is perceived psychosocial support.

It was operationalised in four (4) modalities according to the House model [9] :

- Emotional support ;
- Esteem support
- Information support
- Material support

II. 7.1.3 The dependent variable

According to Mvessomba [38], the dependent variable designates the behaviour that the researcher wants to study or measure, and it is therefore the behaviour that reflects the action of the independent variable.
The dependent variable in this study is quality of life.

III - 7.2 Technical procedures

The aim will be to talk to the inmates about the benefits of the study, while at the same time raising their awareness. Once their consent has been obtained, they will be given a questionnaire. Each questionnaire will be given an anonymous number in order to maintain confidentiality.

II - 7.3. Data collection and statistical analysis

II - 7.3.1 Data collection

Data was collected using a paper-and-pencil questionnaire given to prisoners under the supervision of a prison guard who acted as a guide. The questionnaires were given to the inmates after they had given their consent, according to the schedule of collection days for each ward, once the volunteers had been identified. Some participants completed the questionnaire in our presence, while others gave it back to us after a few days. In most cases, we met the inmates in the main prison yard.

II - 7.3.2. Data capture and statistical analysis

The data was entered simply using Cspro 2013. Data analysis was carried out using SPSS (Version 26) and Jasp on Windows 10. Two types of analysis were used in this study: descriptive analysis and differential analysis.

II - 7.3.2.1 Descriptive analysis

These initial analyses make it possible to describe the results obtained for each of the study variables. To this end, the study presents the descriptive results for the different measurement scales. The analysis will focus on the presentation of the tables, a central tendency index (the mean) and two dispersion indices (the variance and the standard deviation).

II - 7.3.2.2 Differential analysis

Differential analysis was used to verify the study's hypotheses. The choice of statistical processing tools used was dictated by the nature of the data collected and the study hypotheses. To check whether psychosocial support improves prisoners' quality of life, we used simple linear regression analyses. This technique makes it possible to determine the contribution of the various dimensions of psychosocial support to quality of life.

II -8 Ethical considerations

The anonymity and confidentiality of the information collected will be preserved in accordance with law no.° 2020/010 of 20 July 2020, signed by the President of the Republic, which sets out the procedures for collecting statistical data in Cameroon [39].

CHAPTER III
PRESENTATION OF THE STUDY RESULTS

III.1 Breakdown by gender

Table 2: Breakdown of the sample by number and gender

SEX	Frequency	Percent	Valid Percent	Cumulative Percent
male	328	77.910	77.910	77.910
female	93	22.090	22.090	100.000

The table above shows that 328 prisoners interviewed, or 77.91%, were men and 93, or 22.09%, were women.

III.2 Breakdown by age

Table 3: Age distribution of the sample

AGE	Frequency	Percent	Valid Percent	Cumulative Percent
15-20	36	8.551	8.551	8.551
20-25	101	23.990	23.990	32.542
25-30	89	21.140	21.140	53.682
30-35	111	26.366	26.366	80.048
35-40	84	19.952	19.952	100.000

The table above shows that 111 inmates, or 26.3% of our respondents, were aged between 30 and 35.

Table 4: Breakdown of the sample by profession

PROFESSION	Frequency	Percent	Valid Percent	Cumulative Percent
Retailers	109	25.891	25.891	25.891
Civil servants	46	10.926	10.926	36.817
Students	63	14.964	14.964	51.781
Households	54	12.827	12.827	64.608
Small Trades	119	28.266	28.266	92.874
Cultivators	30	7.126	7.126	100.000
ssing	0	0.000		
Total	421	100.000		

The table above shows that 119 prisoners, or 28.2% of our respondents, work in odd jobs.

III.3 Breakdown by religion

Table 5: Breakdown of sample by religion

RELIGION	Frequency	Percent	Valid Percent	Cumulative Percent
Christian	336	79.810	79.810	79.810
Animist	13	3.088	3.088	82.898
3 Muslims	49	11.639	11.639	94.537
4 others	23	5.463	5.463	100.000

The table above shows that the majority of respondents, 336 prisoners or 79.81%, are Christians.

III.4 Breakdown by marital status

Table 6: Breakdown of sample by marital status

MATRIMONIAL	Frequency	Percent	Valid Percent	Cumulative Percent
single,	275	65.321	65.321	65.321
Married	123	29.216	29.216	94.537
divorced,	10	2.375	2.375	96.912
Widows	13	3.088	3.088	100.000

The table above shows that the majority of respondents, 275 prisoners or 65.32%, were single.

III.5 Breakdown by penal status

Table 7: Breakdown of the sample by criminal status

Frequencies for PENAL				
	Frequency	Percent	Valid Percent	Cumulative Percent
Defendants	272	64.608	64.608	64.608
Cassassionate	11	2.613	2.613	67.221
Convicts	103	24.466	24.466	91.686
Callers	35	8.314	8.314	100.000
Missing	0	0.000		
Total	421	100.000		

The table above shows that 272 prisoners, i.e. 64.6% of our respondents, were remand prisoners.

III.6 Breakdown by length of imprisonment

Table 8: Breakdown of the sample by length of incarceration

INCARCERATION	Frequency	Percent	Valid Percent	Cumulative Percent
0-6 months	180	42.755	43.584	43.584
6-1 years	87	20.665	21.065	64.649
1-2 years	70	16.627	16.949	81.598
2-4 years	40	9.501	9.685	91.283
More than 4 years	36	8.551	8.717	100.000

The table above shows that 180 prisoners, or 42% of our respondents, have been in prison for at least 6 months.

III.7 Breakdown by number of children

Table 9: Breakdown of sample by number of children

CHILDREN	Frequency	Percent	Valid Percent	Cumulative Percent
have children	301	71.496	71.496	71.496
do not have children	120	28.504	28.504	100.000

The table above shows that 301 prisoners interviewed, i.e. 71.4%, have children.

III.8 Descriptive analysis results

In this part of the work, the results of the descriptive analyses are presented for each of the study's variables and their modalities. In the present study, quality of life was assessed in four dimensions, namely the physical dimension, the psychological dimension, the social relationship dimension and the environmental dimension, using the WHO (2000) quality of life assessment questionnaire. The results of the analyses of each of these dimensions are presented here.

Descriptive statistics for perceived physical quality of life

Table 10: Descriptive analysis of perceived physical quality of life

	Mean	Std. Deviation	Minimum	Maximum
PH	2.105	0.634	1.000	4.000

The table above shows that the average score for the physical dimension of quality of life perceived by the 421 inmates surveyed was 2.10. This score is below the theoretical average for a 4-point scale. This score is below the theoretical average of a 4-point scale. The dispersion of scores around this average seems low in view of the value of the standard deviation (E-T = 0.63). However, there was a significant difference between the minimum score (min = 1,000) and the maximum score (max = 4,000) recorded on this scale.

Figure 1: Distribution of scores for the physical dimension of perceived quality of life

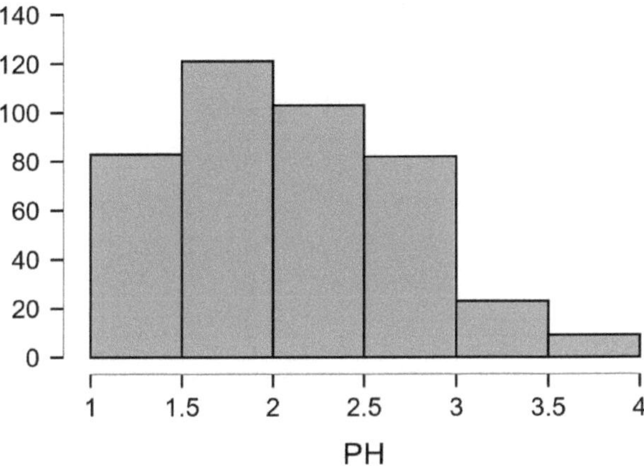

The normal distribution graph seems to show that the scores obtained in the assessment of perceived quality of life are concentrated on the left of the graph.

Descriptive statistics for perceived psychological quality of life

Table 11: Descriptive analysis of perceived psychological quality of life

	MeanStd	. Deviation	Minimum	Maximum
PSY	2.307	0.671	1.000	4.000

This table shows that the average score for the psychological dimension of quality of life perceived by the 421 inmates surveyed was 2.30. This score is slightly higher than the theoretical average for a 4-point scale. This score is slightly higher than the theoretical average on a 4-point scale. The dispersion of scores around this average seems low in view of the value of the standard deviation (S-D = 0.67). However, there was a significant difference between the minimum score (min = 1,000) and the maximum score (max = 4,000) recorded on this scale.

Figure 2: Distribution of scores for the psychological dimension of perceived quality of life

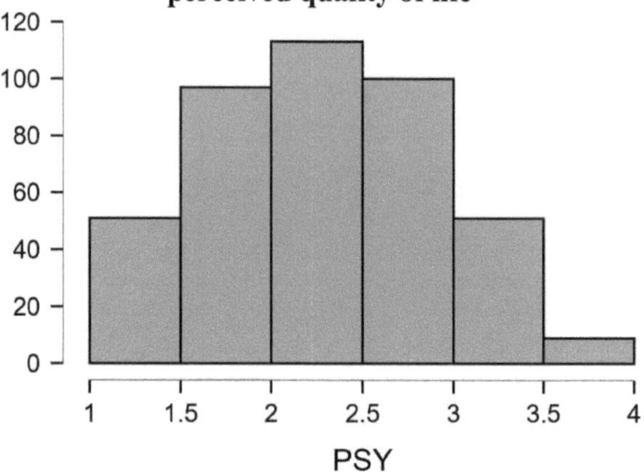

The normal distribution graph seems to show that the scores obtained in the evaluation of the psychological dimension of perceived quality of life are concentrated on the right-hand side of the graph.

Descriptive statistics on quality of life in the perceived social relationship

Table 12: Descriptive analysis of perceived quality of life in social relationships

Mean	Std. Deviation	Minimum	Maximum	
RS	2.055	0.791	1.000	4.000

The table above shows that the mean score for the social relations dimension of the quality of life perceived by the 421 inmates surveyed was 2.05. This score is below the theoretical mean of a 4-point scale. The dispersion of scores around this average seems low in view of the value of the standard deviation (E-T = 0.79). However, there was a significant difference between the minimum score (min = 1,000) and the maximum score (max = 4,000) recorded on this scale.

Figure 3: Distribution of scores for the social relations dimension of perceived quality of life

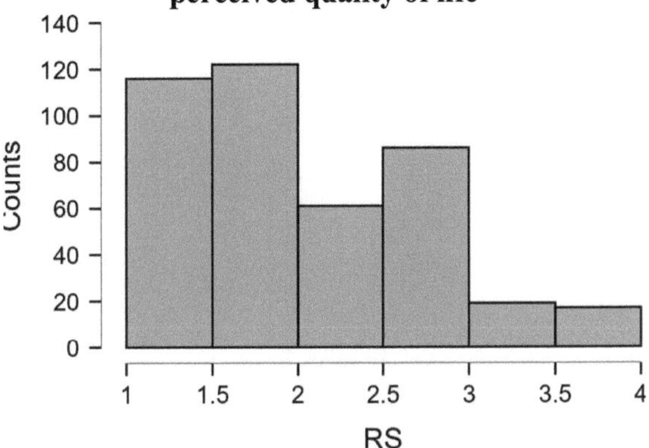

The normal distribution graph seems to show that the scores obtained in the evaluation of the social relations dimension of perceived quality of life are concentrated on the right-hand side of the graph.

Descriptive statistics on perceived environmental quality of life

Table 13: Descriptive analysis of perceived environmental quality of life

	Mean	Std. Deviation	Minimum	Maximum
AT	2.261	0.656	1.000	4.000

The table shows that the average score for the **Environment** dimension of the quality of life perceived by the 421 inmates surveyed was 2.26. This score is below the theoretical average for a 4-point scale. This score is below the theoretical average of a 4-point scale. The dispersion of scores around this average seems low in view of the value of the standard deviation (S-D = 0.65). However, there was a significant difference between the minimum score (min = 1,000) and the maximum score (max = 4,000) recorded on this scale.

Figure 4: Distribution of scores for the environment dimension of perceived quality of life

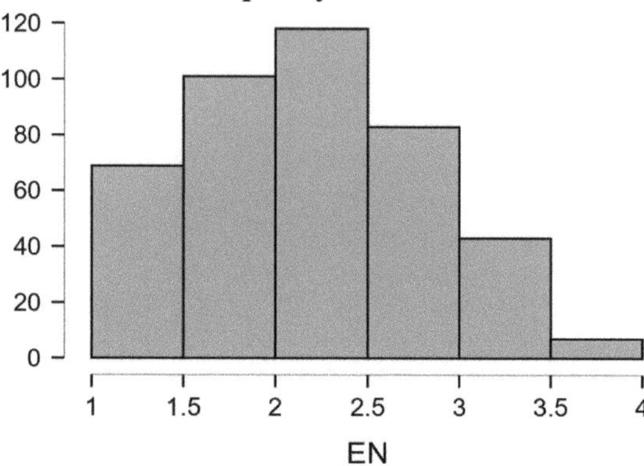

The normal distribution graph seems to show that the scores obtained in the evaluation of the environment dimension of perceived quality of life are concentrated on the right-hand side of the graph.

Descriptive statistics of perceived overall quality of life

Table 14: Descriptive analysis of perceived overall quality of life

	Mean	Std. Deviation	Minimum	Maximum
QLT	2.186	0.552	1.000	3.861

The table above shows that the average score for the overall quality of life perceived by the 421 inmates surveyed was 2.18. This score is below the theoretical average for a 4-point scale. This score is below the theoretical average of a 4-point scale. The dispersion of scores around this average seems low in view of the value of the standard deviation (S-D = 0.55). We note that Nevertheless, there is a significant difference between the minimum score (Min = 1,000) and the score maximum (max = 4,000) recorded on this scale.

Figure 5: Distribution of overall perceived quality of life scores

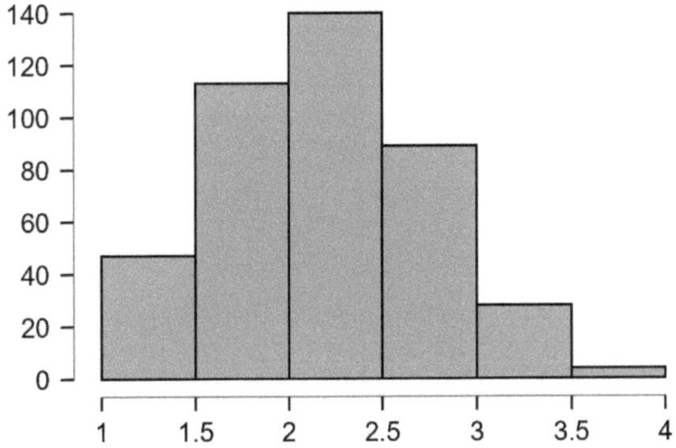

The normal distribution graph seems to show that the scores obtained in the assessment of overall perceived quality of life are concentrated on the left of the graph.

III.9 Results of the descriptive analysis of the dimensions of psychosocial support

In the present study, psychosocial support was assessed along four dimensions, namely emotional support, esteem support, informational support and material support, using the House (1981) model. The results of the analyses of each of these dimensions are presented here.

Descriptive statistics on perceived emotional support

Table 15: Descriptive analysis of perceived emotional support

Mean	Std. Deviation	Minimum	Maximum	
EM	2.181	0.803	1.000	4.000

This table shows that the average score for emotional support perceived by the 421 inmates surveyed was 2.18. This score is below the theoretical average for a 4-point scale. This score is below the theoretical mean of a 4-point scale. The dispersion of scores around this average seems low in view of the value of the standard deviation (E-T = 0.80). However, there was a significant difference between the minimum score (min = 1,000) and the maximum score (max = 4,000) recorded on this scale.

Figure 6: Description of perceived emotional support scores

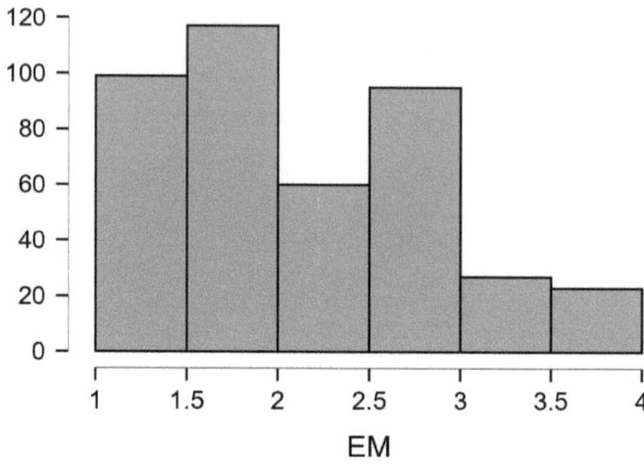

The normal distribution graph seems to show that the scores obtained in the evaluation of perceived emotional support are concentrated on the left of the graph.

Descriptive statistics on perceived esteem support

Table 16: Descriptive analysis of perceived esteem support

Mean	Std. Deviation	Minimum	Maximum	
ES	2.315	0.819	1.000	4.000

The table above shows that the average self-esteem support score for the 421 inmates surveyed was 2.31. This score is below the theoretical average of a 4-point scale. This score is below the theoretical mean of a 4-point scale. The dispersion of scores around this average seems low in view of the value of the standard deviation (S-D = 0.81). However, there was a significant difference between the minimum score (min = 1,000) and the maximum score (max = 4,000) recorded on this scale.

Figure 7: Distribution of perceived esteem support scores

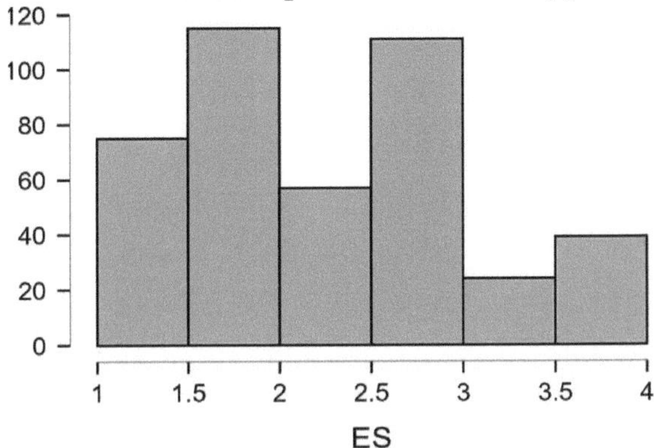

The normal distribution graph seems to show that the scores obtained in the assessment of perceived esteem support are concentrated on the left of the graph.

Descriptive statistics on perceived informational support

Table 17: Descriptive analysis of perceived informational support

Mean	Std. Deviation	Minimum	Maximum	
IN	2.475	0.866	1.000	4.000

This table shows that the average score for informational support perceived by the 421 inmates surveyed was 2.47. This score is below the theoretical average for a 4-point scale. This score is below the theoretical mean of a 4-point scale. The dispersion of scores around this average seems low in view of the value of the standard deviation (S-D = 0.86). However, there was a between the minimum score (Min = 1,000) and the maximum score (max = 4,000) recorded on this scale.

Figure 8: Distribution of perceived informational support scores

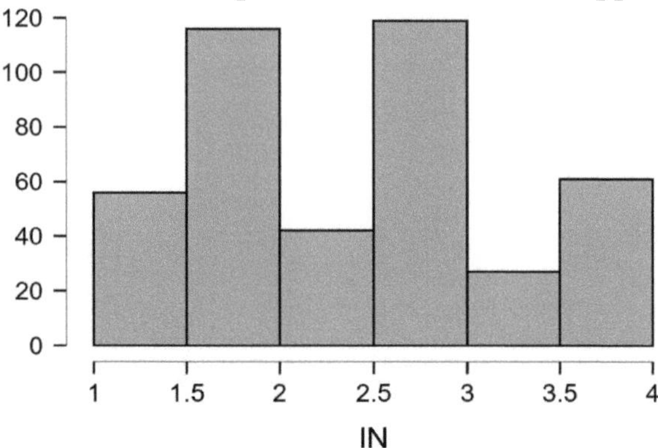

The normal distribution graph seems to show that the scores obtained in the assessment of perceived informational support are concentrated on the left of the graph.

Descriptive statistics on perceived material support

Table 18: Descriptive analysis of perceived material support

Mean	Std. Deviation	Minimum	Maximum	
MA	2.196	0.791	1.000	4.000

This table shows that the average score for material support perceived by the 421 prisoners surveyed was 2.19. This score is below the theoretical average of one 4-point scale. The dispersion of scores around this average seems low in view of the value of the standard deviation (S-D = 0.79). However, there is a significant difference between the minimum score (min = 1,000) and the maximum score (max = 4,000) recorded on this scale.

Figure 9: Distribution of perceived material support scores

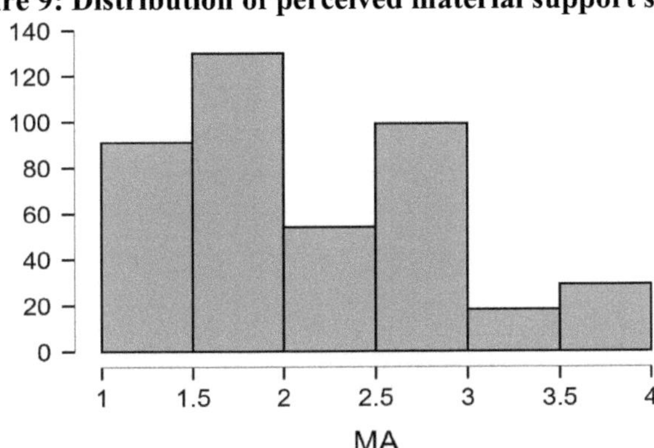

The normal distribution graph seems to show that the scores obtained in the evaluation of perceived material support are concentrated on the left of the graph. A correlational analysis was then carried out between psychosocial support and quality of life. This analysis constitutes the first level of study of the empirical relationship between the two variables.

III.10 Correlation analysis

In the scientific literature, correlation analyses are carried out in order to verify the assumptions prior to the regression analysis. In reality, for To carry out a regression, significant correlation links between the dimensions of the variables must first be obtained. The table below shows the correlation matrix between the dimensions of psychosocial support and those of quality of life for the prisoners surveyed.

Table 19: Correlation matrix

Variable	EM	ES	IN	MA	PH	PSY	RS	AT	QLT
1. EM	-								
2. ES	0.595	-							
	< .001	-							
3. IN	0.386	0.503	-						
	< .001	< .001	-						
4.MA	0.382	0.376	0.530	-					
	< .001	< .001	< .001	-					
5. PH	0.438	0.363	0.314	0.378	-				
	< .001	< .001	< .001		-				
6.PSY	0.335	0.301	0.307	0.292	0.569	-			
< .001									
	< .001	< .001	< .001	< .001	< .001	-			
7. RS	0.481	0.424	0.338	0.391	0.553	0.434	-		
	< .001	< .001	< .001	< .001	< .001	< .001	-		
8. EN	0.499	0.383	0.365	0.412	0.644	0.539	0.520	-	
	< .001	< .001	< .001	< .001	< .001	< .001	< .001	-	
9.QLT	0.533	0.446	0.403	0.450	0.880	0.786	0.738	0.832	-
	< .001	< .001	< .001	< .001	< .001	< .001	< .001	< .001	-

The results of the correlation analysis show that the dimensions of perceived psychosocial support are significantly and positively related to perceived quality of life. Emotional support was significantly and positively related to perceived quality of life (**r= 0.53; p<.001**). However, the value of the correlation coefficient remained moderate. Esteem support maintained a Information support had a significant and positive relationship with perceived quality of life, although the value of the correlation coefficient appeared low (**r= 0.44; p<.001**). Informational support was significantly and positively related to perceived quality of life, although the correlation coefficient appeared low (**r= 0.40; p<.01**). Material support maintained a significant and positive relationship with perceived quality of life, although the value of the correlation coefficient appeared low (**r= 0.45; p<.005**). Simple linear regression analysis gives a better indication of the links between these variables.

III.11 Operational hypothesis verification

This hypothesis was formulated as follows: psychosocial support focusing on emotional support improves the quality of life of prisoners in Douala Central Prison.

III. 11.1 Verification of the first operational hypothesis

This hypothesis was formulated as follows: psychosocial support focusing on perceived emotional support increases the quality of life of inmates at Douala Central Prison.

Table 20: Simple regression of perceived emotional support on quality of life

	R2 adjusted	Beta	T	P
Quality of life	,282		12.89	.001
Emo_Support		,53		

The aim of the analysis presented in the table is to verify the idea that perceived emotional support improves the quality of life of inmates at Douala Central Prison. As both variables (emotional support and quality of life) were measured using numerical scales, the data collected are in the form of continuous scores. We logically chose to use the statistical technique of simple linear least squares regression to carry out this test. The results show that support has a statistically significant influence on prisoners' quality of life (**β= .53; p= .001**). As expected, perceived emotional support in terms of the value of the regression coefficient improved quality of life. The contribution of perceived emotional support in explaining quality of life was almost 28.2% (R^2). This observation is in line with our hypothesis. The $HHHH1$ hypothesis is therefore logically confirmed.

III. 11.2 Verification of the second operational hypothesis

This hypothesis was formulated as follows: psychosocial support focusing on perceived esteem increases the quality of life of prisoners in Douala central prison.

Table 21: Simple regression of perceived esteem support on quality of life

	R2 adjusted	Beta	T	P
Quality of life	,197		10.19	.001
Support_Es		,44		

The objective of the analysis presented in the table is to verify the idea that perceived esteem support improves the quality of life of inmates at Douala Central Prison. As both variables (esteem support and quality of life) were measured using numerical scales, the data collected are in the form of continuous scores. We logically chose to use the statistical technique of simple linear least squares regression to carry out this test. The results show that perceived esteem support has a statistically significant influence on prisoners' quality of life (**β= .44; p=.001**). As might be expected, perceived emotional support in terms of the value of the regression coefficient improved quality of life. The contribution of perceived emotional support in explaining quality of life was nearly 19.2% (R^2). This observation is in line with our hypothesis. Hypothesis H2 is therefore logically confirmed.

III. 11.3 Verification of the third operational hypothesis

This hypothesis was formulated as follows: psychosocial support focusing on informational support improves the quality of life of prisoners in Douala Central Prison.

Table 22: Simple regression of perceived informational support on quality of life

	R2 adjusted	Beta	T	P
Quality of life	.161		9.19	.001
Support_Es		.40		

The objective of the analysis presented in the table is to verify the idea that perceived informational support improves the quality of life of inmates at Douala Central Prison. As both variables (informational support and quality of life) were measured using numerical scales, the data collected are in the form of continuous scores. We logically chose to use the statistical technique of simple linear least squares regression to carry out this test. The results show that perceived esteem support has a statistically significant influence on prisoners' quality of life (**β= .40; p= .001**). As might be expected, perceived informational support in terms of the value of the regression coefficient improved quality of life. The contribution of perceived informational support in explaining quality of life was nearly 16.1% (R^2). This observation is in line with our hypothesis. Hypothesis H3 is therefore logically confirmed.

III. 11.4 Verification of the fourth operational hypothesis

This hypothesis was formulated as follows: psychosocial support focused on material support improves the quality of life of prisoners in Douala Central Prison.

Table 23: Simple regression of perceived material support on quality of life

	R2 adjusted	Beta	T	P
Quality of life	.200		10.30	.001
Support_MA		.45		

The objective of the analysis presented in the table is to verify the idea that perceived material support improves the quality of life of prisoners in Douala Central Prison. As both variables (material support and quality of life) were measured using numerical scales, the data collected are in the form of continuous scores. We logically chose to use the statistical technique of simple linear least squares regression to carry out this test. The results show that perceived esteem support has a statistically significant influence on prisoners' quality of life (**β= .45; p=.001**). As might be expected, perceived informational support in terms of the value of the regression coefficient improved quality of life. The contribution of perceived informational support in explaining quality of life was nearly 20% (R^2_{aj}). This observation is in line with our hypothesis. The *HHHH*4 hypothesis is therefore logically confirmed.Overall, the regression analyses indicate that psychosocial support improves the quality of life of the Douala prison inmates surveyed. However, the linear regression tests implemented analyse the relationship between psychosocial support and quality of life in isolation. To overcome the limitations of this approach, structural equation modelling was chosen. These models are highly accurate, since they take measurement errors into account in all estimation procedures. As a confirmatory statistical method, structural equation modelling can be used to check whether the data collected are consistent with the results obtained. to the theoretical model postulated. In most cases, this theoretical model accounts for a causal explanatory mechanism between the variables studied. The structural model is a combination of all the possible relationships existing between the variables highlighted and their underlying dimensions in the same model.

The validity or otherwise of a structural model is given by structuring indices (TLI, CFI, x2/dll, GFI, NFI, SRMR, NNFI, etc).

III. 12 Results of structural equation modelling

Table 24: Structural equation analysis

Indices	x2/dl	CFI	GFI	TLI	NFI	RMSEA	SRMR
Model	1.99	.96	.99	.91	.91	.07	.04

The results show that the value of the x2/dl ratio (51.824/26) is 1.99. In accordance with the recommendations of Jöreskog and Sörbom (1993), when this value is less than 2, this indicates an excellent fit. This first index indicates that the proposed model provides an adequate representation of the sample data.
The comparative fit index (CFI) derived from the comparison between the proposed model and the null model (in which no link is postulated between the variables) reveals a good level of fit of the model to the data. Its value is very often between 0 and 1, and the higher its value, the better the fit. In this model, the CFI (.96) meets the criterion (.95) of an appreciable fit to the data.
The goodness of fit index (GFI), which is a measure of the fit between the hypothetical model and the observed covariance matrix, has a value of .99. This value meets the criterion of an adequate fit to the data. Also, the Tucker-Lewis Index (TLI) has a value of (.91). This value meets the criterion adequate fit of the data. The normalised fit index (NFI) has a value of .91, indicating an acceptable model fit. The Root Mean Square Error of Approximation (RMSEA) (Steiger, 1990) indicates an acceptable model fit. This value is .07. Note also that the value of the standardised residual root mean square (SRMR) also indicates a good model fit. This value (.04) is less than .08. These structuring indices logically attest to the fact that the model linking psychosocial support to prisoners' quality of life fits the data collected well. Apart from this model fit, the structural equation analysis also reveals that the relationship between quality of life and psychosocial support is very real. Both variables move in the same direction.

Table 25: Regression analysis between psychosocial support and quality of life

VI	VD	Estimate	Std. Error	z-value	P
Support	Quality of life	0.64	0.05	11.15	< .001

As expected, psychosocial support improved the quality of life of the prisoners surveyed **(β= .64; p< .001).** In line with our initial predictions, well-implemented psychosocial support can be a resource for combating precariousness and improving inmates' quality of life. The diagram below illustrates the empirical relationship between psychosocial support and the quality of life of the prisoners surveyed.

Figure 10: Modelling the relationship between psychosocial support and quality of life

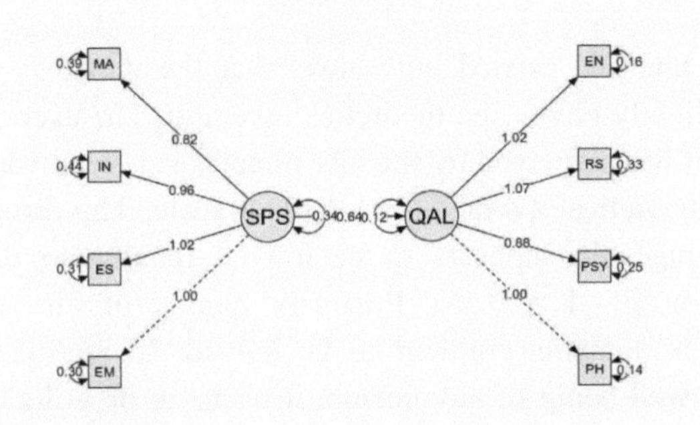

Legend: SPS: psychosocial support; MA: material support; IN: informational support; ES: esteem support; EM: material support; QAL: quality of life; EN: environment; RS: social relationship; PSY: psychological; PH: physical.

CHAPTER IV
DISCUSSION

The aim of this study was to investigate the effect of psychosocial support on the quality of life of inmates at Douala Central Prison. This part of the study provides some answers to this objective. To achieve this objective, we investigated prisoners' social support and quality of life in order to test the following hypotheses

IV.1 Quality of life for inmates at Douala Central Prison

The descriptive analysis carried out shows that the inmates surveyed have a quality of life slightly below the theoretical average. The average score for the overall quality of life perceived by the 421 inmates surveyed was 2.18, which is lower than the theoretical average on a 4-point scale. The dispersion of scores around this average also appears to be low in relation to the value of the standard deviation (E- T = 0.55). Prisoners' quality of life is therefore low, which in itself is a major problem to be solved. In reality, as a necessary resource for the well-being of any person, it wants to be at its best. Only if we stick to the description of the Cameroonian prison environment proposed by (kinombe, 2016) [40], who describes it as a "morgue", can we better justify that the quality of life problems of prisoners require significant investment at all levels.

IV.2 Psychosocial support for inmates at Douala Central Prison

In this study, psychosocial support was studied in four dimensions: emotional support, esteem support, informative support and material support (House, 1981) [39]. The descriptive analysis carried out shows that the inmates of **Douala central prison** who took part in this study appear to report a fairly average level of psychosocial support, across all the dimensions assessed. The indices of central tendency (mean) and dispersion (standard deviation) report the following values: the dimension of emotional support (mean= 2.18; E-T = 0.80), calculated esteem support (mean=2.31; E-T = 0.91), the dimension of psychological support (mean=2.18; E-T = 0.80), the dimension of social support (mean=2.31; E-T = 0.91). informational support (avg= 2.47; E-T = 0.86) and material support (avg= 2.19; E-T = 0.79). It has to be said, therefore, that the inmates interviewed for this study appear to benefit from support, although real for some, but little in the way of mobilising resources to cope with the adversity of the prison environment. In fact, we have made this observation on the basis of our results, since none of the dimensions tested among our respondents is above the theoretical mean of the scale used, which is 2.5. Furthermore, these results are in line with those of MEMONG Fabien et al (2024) [10] in the main prison of Bafia in Cameroon. This gives the impression that the inmates interviewed have been left to their own devices. It might therefore be normal for many of them to be in a state of malaise due to the harsh living conditions and almost non-existent support. We can therefore understand why, in a study by Bausson et al (2012) [41], it emerged that life in a prison environment generates psychological distress in more than 50% of prisoners who lack support. This part of the work is devoted to interpreting and discussing the results obtained from the various hypothesis tests.

- **Emotional support and quality of life**

The first hypothesis of this study was formulated as follows: psychosocial support focusing on perceived emotional support increases the **quality of life** of prisoners in Douala central prison.This hypothesis was confirmed by the results obtained. This indicates that when prisoners perceive good emotional support, their **quality of life** tends to improve. Support helps them to cope, to endure, and to mobilise their adaptive resources, especially in an environment that is recognised as difficult. This support for prisoners is therefore an interesting resource for promoting well-being. In other words, the respondents need emotional support to strengthen their psychological well-being. This demand is hard to meet in a prison system plagued by a shortage of trained health staff working in Cameroon's prisons. In reality, Douala prison has no social worker, let alone a mental health specialist, whose role is essential in providing initial psychological care on entering prison, to help the person cope with the shock of confinement. This support is a powerful stress moderator, and plays a protective role, especially in a context of social isolation such as prison. The person is facing a break with their home environment. They need a professional who will listen and communicate constructively. But unfortunately this is not the case in our prisons. Although humanisation involves listening, speaking, touching and looking, these four concepts are not given much consideration in the treatment of prisoners. The look remains that of surveillance, the touch which is the common denominator is the search, the tone is always threatening and intimidating, (ex inmates of Kondengui 2017).

- **Esteem support and quality of life**

The second hypothesis of this study was formulated as follows: psychosocial support focusing on perceived esteem support increases the **quality of life** of inmates in Douala central prison. This hypothesis was confirmed by the results obtained. This indicates that when prisoners perceive good esteem support, their **quality of life** improves. Psychosocial support focused on perceived esteem support helps to strengthen self-esteem, which is an individual protective factor for mental health, for example. In other words, it plays a major adaptive role in psychological functioning by enabling the individual to adjust to an environment. Psychosocial support focused on boosting the self-esteem of prisoners will enable them to feel recognised and to adopt appropriate behaviour in a variety of situations. It is also a question of reassuring the prisoner about his skills and values. In the context of this study, the results lead us to believe that the inmates of Douala Central Prison do not have activities enabling them to express their skills, with a view to enhancing their self-esteem. According to Valcke (2021), restoring the self-confidence and self-esteem of people who find themselves in prison or who are in a situation of failure and have a rather negative view of themselves means welcoming them by enhancing their skills. [42] According to rule 104 of the Minimum Rules for Imprisonment (2015) [33] prisons are encouraged to set up vocational schools or educational activities that should be given particular attention by the prison administration to enable prisoners to express their skills or acquire new skills with a view to social reintegration after imprisonment. The fact that I did nothing all day long made me feel useless, and I was willing to follow the talks describing the crimes caused by my colloquies," recounts a former Kondengui inmate (2017). A lack of educational activity drowns inmates in idleness, and they can then become interested in exchanging unhealthy experiences that are responsible for recidivism and the resurgence of crime in society.

- **Material support and quality of life**

The third hypothesis of this study was formulated as follows: psychosocial support focused on perceived material support increases the **quality of life** of prisoners in Douala central prison. This hypothesis was confirmed by the results obtained. This indicates that when prisoners perceive good material support, their **quality of life** tends to improve. Material support, whose score appears to be among the lowest in the results (Avg = 2.19; E-T 0.79), is nevertheless the most illustrative of the misery experienced by the inmates surveyed. In fact, in a prison where overcrowding is not a 400% myth, prisoners need substantial material support from third parties to give their lives a little dignity. For most inmates, their family is a "lifeline". immeasurable help in managing the stress caused by the shock of imprisonment. Support during the period of imprisonment helps the prisoner to better manage future events (the shock of being sentenced, the effects of the prison environment, health, nutrition, etc.) and to better adapt to the prison environment.

- **Information support and quality of life**

The fourth hypothesis of this study was formulated as follows: psychosocial support focusing on perceived informative support increases the **quality of life** of prisoners in Douala central prison. The results confirmed this hypothesis. The results of the descriptive analyses revealed that the vast majority of prisoners questioned in this study felt that they did not have good informational support. However, it is useful in that it gives them the means to obtain information about the legal proceedings that concern them, their family and businesses. We think that living without any information about your family and your affairs is no different from being dead. Let's just say that providing information support to a prisoner means enabling him to prepare his defence, his release and his socio-professional reintegration with confidence, while sparing him a great deal of anxiety.

CONCLUSION

Prison conditions in Cameroon inflict a double penalty on inmates. In addition to depriving them of their freedoms, the prison environment deprives prisoners of the enjoyment of all their human rights, including the right to health, food, dignity, privacy, security, equality before the law and the protection of the law, and the presumption of innocence. This situation is responsible for the deterioration in prisoners' quality of life. Faced with this situation, several solutions aimed at protecting this quality of life must be explored to promote the health of people in prisons. Admittedly, the public authorities have not remained silent, as a policy to reduce prison overcrowding has been put in place in our country. However, despite these efforts, prison overcrowding and poor conditions are preventing prisons from fulfilling their regalian role. It is widely accepted that a good psychosocial support network helps to mitigate the secondary effects of criminal conviction and imprisonment. Overall, the results of the study revealed, in line with our hypotheses, that the linear regression analyses carried out revealed that the dimensions of psychosocial support, namely: perceived emotional support **($r = 0.53$; $p < .001$),** perceived esteem support **($r = 0.44$; $p < .001$),** perceived informational support **($r = 0.40$; $p < .01$) and** perceived material support **($r = 0.45$; $p < .005$)** had a statistically significant and positive effect on prisoners' quality of life. These results clearly indicate that these psychosocial support dimensions could be levers in the fight against precariousness and social exclusion. Improve the level quality of quality of life of prisoners in the environment Cameroonian prisons.

.

DIFFICULTIES ENCOUNTERED OUTLOOK

Several limitations should be considered when interpreting and generalising the results of this study. Firstly, the size of the sample (N= 421) suggests modesty in assessing the results obtained, since this proportion is not representative of the reference population. This does not clearly allow us to decide on a better level of consistency between items. This confirms the need to rework our tools to better adapt them to the context. In addition, the measurement tools used in this study were not adapted locally to ensure that they were operational in the context of the study.

SUGGESTIONS

Based on the results of this research, our recommendations mainly concern the organisation of the following activities for prisoners:

- Educational and socio-cultural activities
- Formation of discussion groups during imprisonment with a view to release
- Activities to help prisoners maintain links with their families
- Individual psychosocial interviews
- Workforce development activities
- Home help activities
- Strengthening the management team
- Refresher courses for management staff
- The implementation of statutory controls to inspect conditions of detention
- Generating excitement on social support networks
- Encouraging activities that bring prisoners and their families closer together
- Facilitating visits
- Set up a toll-free number
- Enable convicts to serve their sentences in prisons in their home département

REFERENCES

1) OMCT, SOS-torture 2020 État des lieux du droit à la santé et à la dignité dans les prisons à l'aune de la crise sanitaire en Afrique de l'Ouest et en Afrique centrale, Report of the SOS-Torture Regional Judicial Intervention Group in Africa.

2) Terra, J-L. (2003). Prévention du suicide des personnes détenues - Évaluation des actions misesen mises en place et propositions pour développer un programme complet de prévention. Rapport de mission à la demande du garde des Sceaux, ministre de la Justice et du ministre de la Santé, de la Famille et des Personnes Handicapées.

3) Rizzo & Spitz, (2002) ; influence de la pratique physique sur la qualité de vie en prison : de l'utilisation des activités physiques et sportives comme stratégie d'ajustement spécifique.

4) IARC. (2018). Mental health and psychosocial support. Annual report.

5) Penal Reform International (2015) report global prison trends

6) Minkoa Ngah (2020). Prévalence des facteurs associés à la dépression mentale et à l'anxiété généralisée chez les détenus de la prison centrale de Yaoundé. Doctoral thesis in Psychiatry, University of Yaoundé 1.

7) Christian EYOUM 2023 depression and suicidal ideations among Prisoners of the Douala central prison)

8) GODIN-BLANDEAU (2013) La santé des personnes détenues en France et à l'étranger: une revue de la littérature. Bulletin Epidémiologique Hebdomadaire.

9) HOUSE, J.S. (1981). Work, Stress and Social Support. Addison-Wesley, Reading

10) Memong Ndengue, F. et al (2022). Impact de soutien psychosocial sur la santé mentale des détenus de la prison principale de Bafia. Imjst, Volume 9.

11) DURKHEIM (1897) Le suicide - Etude de sociologie 14th edition Emile Durkheim Serge Paugam

12) Park & Burgess, (1926) Social support and mental health: concept, measures, recent research and implications for clinicians Jean Caron* Stéphane Guay

13) Orford J. (1992) Community Psychology: Theory and Practice. Wiley, Chichester: pp. vii+292. £18.99 ISBN 0-471-93810-6 (paperback)),

14) TARDY C.H. (1985), "Social Support Measurement", American Journal of Community Psychology, vol. 13, n° 2, p. 187-203

15) BARRERA M., (1981). "Social Support in the Adjustment of Pregnant Adolescents: Assessment Issues", in B.H. Gottlieb (ed.), Social Networks and Social Support, Beverly Hills, CA: Sage, pp. 69-96.
16) COHEN S., WILLS T.H. (1985), Stress, social support and the buffering hypothesis, Psychological Bulletin, vol. 98, p. 310-357
17) sabine chiné (2012)

18) (WHO, 2014)..

19) Bruchon-Schweitser (2002),

20) (WHO 1946). [20]

21) Tousignant, M. (1988). Soutien social et santé mentale : une revue de la littérature. Sciences sociales et santé. 6 (1), 77-106.
22) Wade & Kendler, 2000)

23) (Lakey & Cohen, 2000)

24) Boucher and Laprise (2004, p. 118)

25) SHEA and KING-FARLOW, (1976) La qualité de la vie : perspectives théoriques et empiriques Quality of life: theoretical and empirical perspectives Céline Mercier and Jocelyne Filion
26) CARLISLE, E., 1972, The conceptual structure of social indicators in Shonfield, A., Shaw, S., ed, Social Indicators and Social Policy, London, Heinemann Educational Books.

27) BUBOLZ, M., EICHER, J., EVER, J. SONTAG, M. 1980, A human ecological approach to quality of life: Conceptual framework and results of a preliminary study, Social Indicators Research, 7, 103-116
28) REICH, J.W., ZAUTRA, AJ., 1984, Daily event causation: An approach to elderly life quality, Journal of Community Psychology, 12, 312-322'.
29) BIGELOW, D.A., BRODSKY, G., TREWART, L., OLSON, M. 1982,

The concept and measurement of quality of life as a dependent variable in evaluation of mental health services in Stahler, GJ., Tash, W.R., eds, Innovative Approaches to Mental Health Evaluation, New York, Academic Press, 345-366.
30) ABBEY, A., ANDREWS, F.M. 1985, Modeling the psychological determinants of life quality, Social Indicators Research, 16, 1-34
31) (BOUOPDA 2021),

32) Handicap International. (2012). Prison living conditions andpsychological distress of detainees.Collection Recherche et Études Programme Madagascar.
33) Nelson 2015) [33].

34) ACAT (Action by Christians for the Abolition of Torture). (2011, December). Humanisation o f detention conditions in Cameroon.
35) Commission Nationale Consultative Des Droits De L'Homme (2004). Etude sur les droits de l'homme dans la prison htt://www.ladocumentation française.fr/var/storage/rapport Publics (044000133.pdf)
36) code of criminal procedure

37) Myers, A. & Hansen, C.-H. (2007). Experimental Psychology. De Boeck.
38) Mvessomba, A. E. (2016). Pour une psychologie de la santé: une approche psychosociale. L'Harmathan.
39) DECREE N° 92/052OF 27/03/1992 FIXING THE REGIME PENITENTIAIRE AU CAMEROUN (extract
40) (kinombe, 2016) [40]

41) Bausson, M. (2012). Réunir les solitudes, l'exemple d'un projet de Santé mentalecommunautaire au Rwanda. Presses universitaires de France.
42) Valcke (2021) restoring confidence and self-esteem

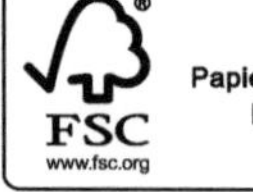

MIX
Papier aus verantwortungsvollen Quellen
Paper from responsible sources
FSC® C105338

Printed by Books on Demand GmbH, Norderstedt / Germany